DIETS TO H

A naturopathic practition
important factor in pso
control can lead to the effective alleviation of the
condition.

DIETS TO HELP

PSORIASIS

HARRY CLEMENTS
N.D., D.O.

THORSONS PUBLISHING GROUP

First published 1981
This revised format edition
first published 1988

British Library Cataloguing in Publication Data

Clements, Harry
Diets to help psoriasis.
1. Psoriasis
2. Diet therapy
I. Title
616.5'26054   RL321

ISBN 0 7225 1758 0

*Published by Thorsons Publishers Limited,
Wellingborough, Northamptonshire, NN8 2RQ, England*

Printed in Great Britain by B. L. & U. Limited,
Wellingborough, Northamptonshire

3   5   7   9   10   8   6   4   2

CONTENTS

It is most unfortunate that most medical men consider psoriasis a hopeless skin condition, for by their pessimistic attitude they discourage a great many patients . . . It is a great mistake, likewise, to emphasize to these patients the chronicity of this disease for the patient easily acquires a definite complex about their condition, and most experts in the treatment of skin disease recognize that this state of mind has a noticeable effect on the course of this disease.

Dr Schwartz

INTRODUCTION

Psoriasis is a chronic skin complaint that causes a great deal of distress among its sufferers. It is characterized by the occurence of dry, reddish patches on the skin which are covered with silvery white scales. The parts of the body most commonly affected are the elbows, knees, scalp, nails and the sacrum region, although in the more severe cases almost the whole of the skin may be involved. It starts as a small reddish papule or pimple. As it develops it takes on a silvery scale which tends to join up with other papules, and thus forming patches of different sizes and shapes. In the early stages it may be difficult to distinguish it from other skin disorders, but the development of the silvery scales characteristic of psoriasis will confirm the diagnosis. The removal of the scales, either by scratching or by other means will lead to what is known as pinpoint bleeding.

In most cases, it is first seen in small patches on the scalp, or on the elbows or the knees, and sometimes at the lower back over the sacrum. Fortunately, the face is very rarely affected, and this is generally supposed to be due to its constant exposure to the sun and air. In a number of cases the complaint may affect the nails of the hands and the toes may lead to their loosening and discoloration. In severe chronic cases, few parts of the outer body may be exempt from the effects of the trouble.

Various types of psoriasis have been described by medical authorities, but these are of more interest to the researchers than to the ordinary sufferer. However, there is a type of popular interest that is associated with arthritis and is said to occur in about ten per cent of all cases. As with rheumatoid arthritis, joints become swollen and painful, especially those of the hands, fingers and the feet, with women as the most frequent sufferers.

Psoriasis is not seen in very early life, possibly appearing at the age of three or four years at the earliest. The young adult seems to be the most susceptible, although it can develop much later in life. It represents about four per cent of all skin diseases, and estimates from the U.S. puts the figure around seven or eight million, which would be about two per cent of the whole population—making it an unsolved medical problem of considerable proportions.

The background to psoriasis is very interesting and does have some bearing on the present attitude towards it. In earlier times it had the misfortune to be associated in the public mind with leprosy and syphilis which added to the problem. In the early years of the nineteenth century, an observant medical man was able to dispel this assumption, and to put the complaint in its proper perspective. At the same time it was shown that psoriasis is a non-contagious complaint, but such preconceived ideas, as with other forms of disease, die hard and even at the present time the question of contagion still occasionally arises.

The disfigurement of the skin which occurs in very severe cases makes the condition very hard to bear; the sufferer finds himself or herself constantly reminded of the existence of the complaint, through its visual manifestation, and there is no doubt that this adds to the problem in the psychological sense. This may tend to make the patient refuse to lead a normal life and to develop a pessimistic outlook—an attitude which must be discouraged at all costs. The fact that many medical authorities say that there is no cure for the disease should be seen in its proper context, as one chronic disease amongst many for which an outright cure is not thought medically possible—for example arthritis, diabetes and coronary disease.

'Psoriasis, as one might expect, has been subjected to many different forms of treatment, and it is true to say that medical and folklore remedies have been used in abundance. Both the intractable nature of the complaint, and the desire for help on the part of the patient, has added to the urge to find palliative measures. Tar and its derivatives have extensibly been used in treatment over the years; x-ray and ultraviolet light therapy have found favour in some cases, and as would be expected new drugs have been developed for use against this complaint. But their uses as palliatives are, of course, limited by their possible side-effects.

Psoriasis, being classified as a skin disease, has led to almost the exclusive use of external remedies in its treatment. From this standpoint it is assumed the complaint affects only the skin and that no other function of the body is involved. That is why we find in medical literature relating to psoriasis very little reference to the state of the general health and nutrition. Indeed, in some cases it is denied that food and nutrition play any part in the disease at all.

The skin is not, of course, just the outer covering of

the body and unrelated to all the other parts and functions. It is one of the most important eliminative systems and is richly supplied with blood vessels and blood and nerves for the carrying out of this vital function. It shares in many other functions of the system and is responsive to internal conditions. A normally functioning skin is a good indicator of sound health and well-being, just as it is a reliable index of changes taking place in the body in cases of disease. From this viewpoint, proper food and sound nutrition which waits upon it is of vital importance in maintaining and restoring the health of the skin, and this is just as true for psoriasis as it is of other skin complaints. In the following pages I plan to show how diet may be used to the best advantage in the management of this widespread and distressing skin disorder.

1
ADOPTING A DIET

In adopting a diet for a condition like psoriasis its success will depend on its adjustment to the special needs of the particular individual, and the intelligent co-operation of the sufferer is essential in achieving this object. It is not just a matter of selecting foods for their food values—protein, carbohydrates, fats, vitamins and so on—for foods produce varying reactions in different people and this fact is particularly applicable in any person suffering from a disease-reaction like psoriasis. The old adage 'one man's meat is another man's poison' is very appropriate here. Today, we speak of it as allergy, in which foods or parts of foods may produce an adverse reaction in the bodily system and thus contribute to a particular complaint. A number of foods have been identified in this respect, among them may be mentioned wheat, chocolate, eggs, oranges and so on. The fact is, that as long as these food sustances are included in the diet of a susceptible person, these adverse reactions will occur.

Environmental Factors
A very important aspect of the allergic effects of certain foods is that the discovery can only be made through trial and error. As a consequence, the

individual must be willing to take an active part in the procedure. While this may seem to be more troublesome than just being 'put on a diet', the fact is, that unless such a food allergen can be identified (provided of course, that it does exist), the success of the diet may be very doubtful.

Another point that must be considered when adopting a diet for a complaint like psoriasis, so far as the kind of food is concerned, is the family background. Most authorities when dealing with this complaint ascribe its cause, in part, to a dominant gene and this hereditary factor may in some degree depress both the sufferer and those who treat it. But we should remember that genes and the environment are not separate: they operate together. So, it is to the environment and, in particular, the food we take in from our environment, to which we should address our efforts for its improvement.

Many of those who suffer from psoriasis can look back over years of food and feeding habits and other environmental factors, which have not been radically changed, and it may well be that one or more members of the family have suffered in the same way, which may give rise to the thought that heredity has played a part in the trouble. But one should remember that the same means tend to produce the same ends. What is required is a radical departure from the diet and dietetic habits which have persisted in the family for so many years, and which have tended to undermine the bodily health and resistance and to perpetuate the weakness.

The reason for the adoption of a specific diet for a complaint such as psoriasis must go beyond that of taste and the satisfaction of hunger. It must concern us with making radical change in the chemistry of the body: the balance between the acid/alkaline reaction of the bodily system must be a first priority with a curative diet. While, in this respect, adequate and suitable food is essential, it is its final incorporation into the system that is the real test of its value, which is a matter of efficient digestion and assimilation. In a sense, the breaking down, digesting and assimilation of food is a relatively simple process, and many people are under the impression that if food does not immediately disagree with them it must, therefore, be suitable. But it is in the utilization of the nutriment by the millions of cells in the body that is the keynote in good nutrition. As a matter of fact, a diet of refined, conventional foods that may be deficient in some of the ingredients essential to sound nutrition, may place very little strain on the digestive organs and processes, and thus deceive the person into thinking that all is well with his digestion and nutrition.

Sound, Wholefood Diet

A refined diet may be deficient in all the vital elements which are only to be found in the more natural foods, and for this reason more of such foods must be included in the menus. This means also that as many foods as possible must be taken in as nearly as possible their natural state. This means that free use must be made of fresh raw salads, raw vegetables and raw ripe fruit, together with properly cooked whole vegetables and foods like whole grains, such as wheat, oats, rice and so on. Unlike the refined and over-concentrated foods (the so-called convenience foods), these natural foods contain all the essential vitamins, minerals and other elements in the most suitable proportions for the promotion of sound nutrition so necessary for normal health and recovery from illness.

It is true that in recent years these ideas have been more generally accepted, so that many people have improved their diet in this way. But the vital part which these foods play in the management of the various complaints have not been sufficiently stressed, mainly, of course, because people turn to the use of medicines at such times and the benefits of a properly regulated diet is overlooked. Indeed, in skin complaints, particularly in one like psoriasis, it is often stated that there is no scientific proof that diet plays a significant part. Such a negative attitude is often very discouraging to the sufferer.

If we have to wait for scientific proof in such matters we may have to wait for a very long time and many sufferers may be deprived of real help in the meantime. From much practical experience over a good many years, I can confirm the fact that a carefully adjusted diet, consisting of a generous amount of the natural foods, with allergenic ones eliminated, will prove to be the most effective form of treatment. It seems to me to be only commonsense to argue that sound nutrition, based on suitable food, should be given first priority both in health and disease.

Toxin-free, Low Protein Diet
Of course, some patients who suffer from a complaint like psoriasis (which seems to be peculiar to their own physical and mental make-up) may have to limit themselves to foods which appear to be most suitable to their own case. In this respect experience has shown that it is better, if possible, to avoid the use

of animal flesh and fish; these foods are more likely to produce toxins within the system and thus aggravate the condition. Those who have to deprive themselves in this way need not fear inadequate nutrition. Many people prefer to live on a fleshless diet and have enjoyed good health as a result. It is generally assumed, of course, that the omission of it from the diet might lead to protein deficiency, but if wholefoods are included in the menus, together with whole grains and the legumes, there is no danger of that happening, especially if animal products such as milk, cheese and eggs are included.

As a matter of fact, experience has clearly shown that sufferers from psoriasis should follow a relatively low protein diet, and avoiding the use of meat and meat products is the best way of doing so. In any case, too free use is made of these foods by many people and this tends to lead to poor elimination and consequently poor health. The adoption of a diet that is far more generous in the use of the fruit and vegetables and other natural foods will be the best way to overcome the sluggish action of the bowels from which many psoriasis patients suffer. Overcoming the trouble in this way is very much better than the use of the laxative drugs, which merely palliate the condition.

Summary
These are all important ideas that the patient should think about when adopting a diet for psoriasis: to watch for foods which may cause allergic reactions; to make use of the whole natural foods as much as possible; to avoid the use of the refined and extracted foods like white sugar; white flour and the products made from them; to avoid, or be extremely moderate

with the flesh foods, and to keep the protein foods on the low side.

In setting out the practical dietetic instruction for the management of the complaint all these important matters will be taken into consideration, and an understanding of the importance of them by the sufferer will no doubt make the treatment more fruitful.

2

THE FOUR-WEEK TREATMENT PLAN

In the dietary management of psoriasis a radical change of food and food habits is usually necessary. This calls for a preliminary period in which the new changes and ideas are gradually introduced. It may be conveniently divided up into four weekly periods. The first one is perhaps the most difficult since it tests the self-discipline of the individual and his willingness to co-operate in putting the new ideas into practice. In the first week of the treatment the idea is to increase the eliminating functions of the body, and thus rid it of the toxins. These may exist as a result of the previous unsuitable diet in which, in a great many cases, the excessive use of meat and other high protein foods have tended to overload the system. As a rule, when the changes and the testing time of the first week have been carried out, the rest of the treatment will be more easily and pleasantly accomplished.

FIRST WEEK

Day 1
This should be a fast day in which no solid food should be taken. Hunger should be satisfied with generous amounts of fruit juices of various kinds—orange, grapefruit, apple, pineapple. A hot

lemonade made with a little honey, if desired, may be taken or a cup of weak tea if taken with a little milk but no sweetening.

Day 2 and 3

A cup of weak tea without sweetening may be taken before breakfast if desired.

Three meals of fruit only should be taken each day chosen from the following list: apples, oranges, grapefruit, pears, bananas, melon, tomatoes, plums, dates, sultanas, peaches, raspberries, strawberries, blackberries, figs and grapes. At least three of them should be taken at each meal so that in the course of the two days practically all of them will have been included. It is important to make use whenever possible of the fruits in season so as to take advantage of their freshness.

Days 4-8

Breakfast: Fruit only, as chosen on the previous day.

Midday   A salad made up of all kinds of raw
meals: vegetables chosen from the following list: lettuce, white cabbage, carrot, cucumber, courgette, watercress, mustard, cress, tomatoes, celery, radish, spring onions, parsley. (As with fruit, in the course of the meals the whole of the list of vegetables should be included in the menus.) Prepare the salad dressing by mixing together lemon juice, vegetable oil and sea salt, and adding to it the finely chopped parsley and spring onions.

Evening meals: This meal should consist of cooked vegetables chosen from the following list: potatoes, carrots, parsnips, cauliflower, cabbage, onions, spinach, turnips, celery, peas, string beans, broccoli, courgettes, artichokes. Three or four of these vegetables should be taken at each meal, preferably baked, steamed or pressure-cooked (when suitable). You should certainly never cook them in salted water or discard any water you might use in cooking. Parsley sauce (not cheese sauce) or yeast gravy may be added if desired.

If it is more desirable, the midday and evening mealtimes may be reversed. In many cases the effect of the week's dieting will make itself shown in the improved function of the bowel and lightening of the colour of the urine and the stools.

SECOND WEEK

On rising: Unsweetened weak tea or hot lemon drink.

Breakfast: Fruit only, as in the first week.

Midday meals: Salad, as in in first week. Carbohydrate food, such as wholewheat bread or wholewheat products, or a rice or potato dish may be added.

Evening meals: As in the first week, to which may be added an omelette or other egg dish or cottage or hard cheese.

At the end of the week a look back over the two weeks of dieting should be made. What effect has it had on the digestion and elimination? Has there been an increase in flatulence? Did any food appear to upset the digestion? Did you develop any kind of aversion to any of the foods? If so, omit them from the diet—there are plenty of others to choose from. With a radical change of diet (which this may mean), you may experience temporary changes in your digestive functions.

THIRD WEEK

On rising:	Weak tea unsweetened or hot lemon.
Breakfast:	One kind of fruit, preferably grapes or apples. A glass of milk or yogurt.
Midday meals:	Lettuce and tomatoes with cream cheese. Wholewheat bread and butter.
Evening meals:	Baked potato with a little butter. Green peas, carrots. Baked apple or stewed figs or prunes.

During this week the number of fruits and vegetables have been restricted. The diet up to the third week has been definitely on the alkaline side and its effect on the symptons of the complaint may be noticed.

FOURTH WEEK

On rising:	Unsweetened tea or hot lemon drink.
Breakfast:	Fruit of personal choice. Muesli with milk, or wholewheat product of personal choice.

Midday meal: Salad made with a selection of all your favourite raw vegetables dressed with lemon juice, vegetable óil and sea salt, or home-made mayonnaise. Baked potato with butter. Banana and other dried fruit such as dates and figs if desired.

Evening meals: Two or three cooked vegetables of personal choice with an omelette or poached or scrambled eggs. Baked apple or stewed figs or prunes with cream.

Why Diet Treatment?

The four weeks of the diet treatment, if carried out carefully and conscientiously, will probably have changed the sufferer's attitude towards food and nutrition. Particularly, of course, if his eating habits in the past have been of the most conventional kind. It may, therefore, be in place to consider some of the reasons for the change and how it may help in dealing with this intractible complaint.

Up to now the individual has probably been in the habit of thinking that the cure of the complaint lies in external applications, regarding it as a local disorder of the skin. This, of course, is in accordance with common thinking in the matter.

Diet treatment is based on a very different conception of the trouble. It is assumed that it is a constitutional complaint in which many different functions of the body are involved; in particular the eliminative functions of the system which is shared by the bowel, the kidneys, the lungs and the skin. Now, it is very easy to understand that elimination is a very important function of the body. There is a constant building-up and breaking-down process going on in the system with the production of waste products which have to be removed from the body. Failure in this respect, or, indeed just a slowing down of this function, is certain to have adverse effects upon the whole body and possibly on the mental processes.

It is known that diet plays a very important part in all the eliminative processes, and Nature Cure in particular, has always stressed this fact. It is known also that the more whole natural foods that are included in the diet the more effective the eliminative processes will be. These foods, carrying with them fibre and other natural activating substances, provide the stimulus so necessary to elimination, and this is the reason for the use of the raw salad, conservatively cooked foods and whole grains. On the other hand, the flesh foods and the refined ones like white flour and sugar, so commonly in use, tend to depress the eliminative process while at the same time add toxic substances to the system.

The ordinary person when thinking about elimination usually regards the bowel function as the important one—in some cases the only one. It is, of course, very important, but unlike the other eliminative processes through the lungs, kidneys and the skin it is not directly concerned with the blood stream. The food tube runs right through the body and the food taken into it is acted upon by the digestive juices so that it is ready for absorption. The residue is left for elimination from the large intestine or the bowel.

The normal passage of food and waste through the tube is very important in the maintenance of health and in the treatment of all forms of illness. The composition of the food will determine to a great extent the eliminative function of the bowel. If it is composed of mainly the natural foods, in which the so-called roughage is included, the passasge of the food through the tube will be taken at a normal pace and the resulting waste will be removed in the same manner. If, on the other hand, the diet is composed mainly of animal products, together with a generous amount of the refined, over-concentrated and the convenience foods, the whole process will be considerably retarded and the waste material retained for prolonged periods, resulting in constipation.

In recent times constipation has been held responsible for many forms of illnessess including diverticulitis and even cancer, and apart from such local troubles there is no doubt that it may play a major part in causing many other complaints affecting the kidneys, the chest and the skin. It is generally recognized by many medical authorities that it is a condition usually accompanying psoriasis—a fact which I can confirm from experience in treating the complaint.

Such a condition cannot be properly treated with laxative drugs; indeed, their use may be counter-productive. The diet must be of an eliminative nature, and this is why the four-week treatment plan is so important. There is little doubt that, if it is carefully carried out the most significant progress toward recovery will have been made.

Observe the Effects

The sufferer might now take stock of the effects of the treatment, not only on the condition of the skin, but also of its effects on his general health and well-being. Has the general feeling of health been affected in any way? What about minor ailments from which may have arisen in the past? If there has been a tendency to catarrh and colds, has this improved in any way? What about headaches? Many people who suffer in a minor way in this respect are inclined to put up with them or take an occasional aspirin or similar remedy for relief. Has the diet helped to give relief? What about the digestion? If there has been in the past digestive troubles with perhaps heartburn, has this responded to the new diet? Has a change been noted in the action of the bowel and the flow of the urine, both of which are to be expected on a more eliminative diet.

If no trouble has been experienced with the various foods used, one may reasonably expect that no allergen has been operating. If, on the other hand, a particular kind of food has been discarded because of digestive upset, it is a good plan to use it exclusively at two or three meals and watch the effects. It must not be forgotten, however, that there can be an interaction between foods as there is between drugs. Recently, drug interactions have become an important feature of medical research since combinations of drugs may induce unexpected side-effects. The same thing may happen with the various foods and this point should be kept in mind when a particular food appears to be associated with disordered digestion. There is no doubt that certain combinations of foods throw less strain in the digestive organs and this point will be dealt with later on.

3
THE BASIC DIET

Having carried out the four-week treatment plan, the sufferer should now think about planning a basic diet that should form his general mode of food and food habits. It should be said, however, that in severe cases of the complaint the four-week treatment plan may have to be carried out twice, or even more times to get the complaint under control. But, in each case, a month or so should be spent on the basic diet in between such sessions. If, through certain circumstances, such as travelling or some other situation you have had to use less suitable food, re-adopting the four-week plan would be a very desirable preventive measure.

Ordinarily, most people take three meals a day and this order will be observed in planning the basic diet. Meals taken in this way allow for enough time to elapse between each meal so that the digestive process may be carried out. On the other hand, there need not be any firm and fast rule about the number of meals taken during the day. A number of people may find that two meals may be more conducive to good digestion; indeed, in the United States some years ago Dr Dewey used this plan in the treatment of his patients and claimed many successful results. It was called the no-breakfast plan; in such an affluent country where there is much overfeeding and illnesses associated with it, a plan like this might well serve a very useful purpose.

Ensuring a Balanced Diet

For most practical purposes, however, the three-meals-a-day plan is probably the best arrangement for the ordinary person. It has the advantage of bringing a certain order into dietary habits and allows for a greater number of foods to be brought into the menus; and the greater the number of foods, the greater the number of complementary combinations that are possible, it enables one for example, to use a preponderance of fruits at one meal in combination with other suitable articles of food. At the next meal raw salads can form the basis and at the following meal cooked vegetables can predominate. This scheme has many advantages. It makes sure that not only is each meal more likely to be well balanced, but it means also that all the food taken over the whole day is properly balanced. This is far better than the conventional way of just taking foods in a haphazard manner—just adding here and there the various articles of diet with no regard for balanced nutrition. Another important point is that it gives priority to the whole, natural fruits and vegetables which are the best source of vitamins and minerals. It reverses the usual order of foods and revokes the view held by many people that these foods are merely trimmings to a meal.

In stressing the importance of these foods in this way it means that not only will more attention be paid to their use but a new interest will develop in the number that can and should be used. Fruits and vegetables vary very considerably in their vitamin and mineral content and in order to ensure a proper supply of essential nutrients, a sufficient quantity of these foods must be used. This is particularly important in all forms of illness, and in chronic complaints like psoriasis it is imperative that all the essential elements are included in the diet.

Another important point in connection with this arrangement of the diet is that it tends to limit the use of the protein and the carbohydrate foods which are so often used in excess. If room has to be made for the fruit, salads and cooked vegetablés as the essential and dominant part of the meal, less emphasis will be laid on the protein and carbohydrate foods, and this will certainly be to the benefit of the patient. The limitation of protein foods, in particular, is something which the sufferer must face if the complaint is to be kept under control. This especially applies, of course, to animal protein.

A Report of Success

It may encourage sufferers to know that at least one doctor made use of a low protein diet in the treatment of psoriasis and with considerable success. Some years ago, Dr L. D. Bulkley of New York, after many years of such practice made the following report.

> The cutting off of the supply of animal protein foods has been very remarkable and striking in many instances. Patients continually notice the change in the colour and character of the eruption, it paling and becoming less scaly, and even entirely disappearing in some weeks with absolutely no local treatment. . . . There have been a number of patients who have faithfully pursued the plan of treatment, in whom a long-existing psoriasis has remained absent, and who, having become accustomed to the diet, say they have lost the desire for flesh food and will not touch it again.

It is unfortunate that such reports seem to make no impact on general medical opinion which seems to give so little attention to the diet and nutritional factor in the treatment of this complaint. Indeed, some adopt a quite irrational attitude and deny any relationship at all. If we go without food over a prolonged period we die; if we live on deficiency food we suffer from deficiency diseases; if we overeat, we suffer from obesity or other complaints. It seems only reasonable to argue that when the body is going through the crisis of any illness it needs every essential nutritional aid to assist in its recovery.

A Week's Basic Diet

Let us see now how the foregoing ideas can be applied in arranging a week's basic diet. First of all, we should give some thought to the nature of the meals in relation to the condition of the body and the physical and mental activities of the individual.

Breakfast

In this respect the first meal of the day is very important. Most people take food three to four hours before retiring and the sleeping period is about eight hours so that at breakfast time, with reasonably normal digestion, the stomach will be devoid of food. During sleep the membranes of the alimentary tract, its inner lining, tend to secrete toxic wastes into the stomach and the bowels; people who suffer from catarrh know how it accumulates during the night to be released in the morning.

There is no doubt that raw fresh fruit is of optimum value when taken at breakfast time. Its acids and fibres have a stimulating and cleansing effect on the membranes of the digestive organs, hastening the passage of the waste materials and, at the same time, supplying the system with vitamins and minerals when absorption of them is best achieved. For some people, a breakfast meal of the fresh fruits, with the addition of dried ones is satisfying enough the whole year around, but others may find, especially in the cold weather that they need extra food in the form of carbohydrates or milk. However, in cases where these foods are added, the fresh fruit should be of fairly generous quantity and always taken in the first part of the meal.

Lunch

Lunch, it should be noted, is usually taken at a time when the physical or mental activity is at full stretch and using up a great deal of nervous energy. In consequence, as little of the energy as possible should be expended in the digestion of food and, contrary to general opinion, a salad of tender raw vegetables is far better in this respect than the commonly used cooked food. For that reason it should form the major part of the meal and, as with fruit, the first part of it. The addition of some carbohydrate foods make an ideal arrangement for those who would desire to feel fresh and alert during the whole day.

Evening Meal

The evening meal is the leisurely one, and is undoubtedly the best time for the cooked foods. The relaxation period of the day has set in and full advantage should be taken of it—before the meal, during it and after it. The foods taken at this meal should be the ones that are more suitable when cooked, and there are, of course, quite a number of them. Potatoes, root, and some other vegetables come within this category; the same is true of some animal products, particularly meat and fish if they are used. It is a mistake to use articles made of sugar and fat, pastries and so on; it is far wiser, if one wishes to get a good night's sleep, to take a baked apple or a similar fruit dish as they are far more easily digested. Again, as against common practice, the fruit should be taken as the first part of the meal.

BASIC DIET:
MENUS FOR SEVEN DAYS

Day 1

Breakfast: Fresh and dried fruit only.

Lunch: Salad of tomatoes, cucumber and lettuce, dressed with lemon juice, vegetable oil and sea salt. Rye crispbread and butter.

Evening meal: Baked apple. Cooked potatoes, carrots and peas. Grated Cheddar cheese.

Day 2

Breakfast: Fresh and dried fruit. Yogurt.

Lunch: Watercress, avocado and tomatoes with cottage cheese. Wholewheat or rye crispbread with butter.

Evening meal: Grapefruit. Baked potatoes, cooked spinach and omelette.

Day 3

Breakfast: Fresh and dried fruit. Wholewheat toast with butter.

Lunch: Salad or shredded or chopped white cabbage, red or green pepper and celery, dressed with mayonnaise. Rye crispbread with butter.

Evening
meal: Grapes. Brown rice dish with courgette
                 and onions.

Day 4

Breakfast: Fresh and dried fruit. Bowl of rolled oat
                 porridge.

Lunch: Chicory, grated carrots, spring onions,
                 radishes. Dressed with lemon juice,
                 vegetable oil and sea salt.

Evening
meal: Melon. Baked potatoes, baked onions
                 and courgette. Grated Cheddar cheese.

Day 5

Breakfast: Fresh and dried fruit. Muesli with milk
                 or yogurt.

Lunch: Celery and grated carrots. Chop finely
                 parsley and spring onions and add to
                 lemon juice, vegetable oil and sea salt
                 and use as dressing. Rye crispbread with
                 butter.

Evening
meal: Peaches. Baked potatoes, cauliflower
                 and parsley sauce. Poached egg.

Day 6

Breakfast: Fresh and dried fruit. Shredded Wheat
                 with milk.

Lunch: Tomatoes, lettuce, sliced beetroot. Add
                 dressing as made for fifth day.

Evening
meal: Vegetable soup. Baked potatoes with
                 carrots and peas or broad beans or
                 string beans. Cheddar cheese.

Day 7

Breakfast: Fresh and dried fruit. Yogurt or a little cottage cheese.

Lunch: Avocado, lettuce and mustard and cress. Dress with home-made mayonnaise. Wholewheat bread and butter.

Evening meal: Stewed prunes. Boiled potatoes in their skins with brussels sprouts and courgettes. Scrambled eggs.

The seven-days menus should follow the four-week treatment plan. Some variation may be made in them providing the main pattern is observed. Advantage should, of course, always be taken of the fresh and seasonal fruits and vegetables that come into the market or are obtainable from the garden. Individual taste comes into the matter and no doubt some of the meals maybe more liked than others; in future menus devised by the individual, favourite dishes can, of course, be included more often.

Avoiding Toxins
It will be noted that in the menus the refined, over-concentrated convenience foods have been carefully excluded. It is well known that the skin is very sensitive to any toxic substance taken into the system; many of the side-effects of drugs are shown in a reaction of the skin in the form of eruptions and whenever they occur search should be made for the foreign substances that may have been used. In the preparation of the refined and convenience foods, white sugar, white flour and many preservatives and other additives have to be employed. The number of artificial additives in use runs into the thousands and

while the authorities endeavour to make them as safe as possible, no one can possibly tell what the individual reaction to them may be. It has been learned by long and sad experience that no drug is totally safe nor can its reaction in every individual be accurately predicted. This is true of every foreign substance that may be used in the preparation of the various foodstuffs.

We cannot, of course, when living in an industrial society completely safeguard ourselves from these substances, but we can go a good way in their avoidance by making as much use as possible of the whole natural foods, especially if they are used as nearly as possible in their natural state. While this is important for everyone, it is of paramount importance to those suffering from skin problems and particularly for those plagued by psoriasis. Of course, the modern way of living does make it more and more difficult to produce your own wholesome food. For those who do have gardens, and the will and energy to cultivate them, such foods would make a real contribution towards their health and wellbeing.

We cannot emphasize too strongly that the sufferer from psoriasis must, when arranging future menus, include in them a generous amount of the whole natural foods.

4

HEALTHFOOD HINTS FOR PSORIASIS

Centuries ago, Hippocrates, known as the Father of Medicine, told us that food is the best remedy. But clearly food must be of good quality and proper quantity if it is to fulfil such a purpose. Of course, in the strict sense of the term, food is not a remedy—it is a necessity. It is essential for maintenance of health and resistance to illness, and as a supplement to the curative power of the body in recovery from disease. From this viewpoint its importance and significance in all forms of ill-health cannot be over-estimated.

Develop the Right Eating Habits

But having gone to the trouble of getting good and proper food we must make sure that we do not lose its benefits through bad eating habits. Most people eat in a haphazard way giving little thought to the nutritional value of food and its consequences within the bodily system. Excessive drinking of tea and coffee and indiscriminate use of fat and sugar is undulged in without fully understanding that it may undermine health. Some people are beginning to see the relationship between these habits and heart disease, but priority should be given to them in all forms of complaints, including, of course, psoriasis.

In the proper use of food we should remind ourselves of some elementary facts. Few people eat from real hunger: they eat because of the time and the serving of the meal. The appetite is coaxed by over-sweetened and spiced foods and condiments, by-passing, as it were the instinctive reactions of the body. This results in over-eating which is widespread in societies where refined and packaged foods form the major part of the diet. Such a diet makes itself known in many ways. It is largely responsible for the coated tongue, frequent bouts of colds and catarrh, the dull headaches and the heavy feeling when getting up in the morning and the inability to 'get going' with the daily tasks.

So, the individual must be willing to develop good eating habits and be respectful of his bodily needs. Eating when there is no relish for food is an imposition that will yield very little beneficial results. Over-eating leads to over-loading and over-working of the digestive organs, with consequent drain on the vital energy and nervous system, and the continuance of present complaints and the promotion of future ones. Enough time should be given between meals to allow the stomach to empty and so be prepared to receive the next meal. When physically or mentally exhausted it is better to postpone the next meal for a while, to allow the body much-needed rest. Also eating a meal too quickly will prevent proper mastication of the food. Treated in this manner the soft carbohydrate foods will not be thoroughly mixed with the saliva, and this may lead to fermentation in the stomach and flatulence. Stress of all kinds adversely affects the processes of digestion, and the assimilation of food, and lowers the resistance to illness. The effect of excessive stress on the heart and circulation is well recognized today, but it is just as operative in many other complaints including psoriasis.

Selecting Good Food

The part played by the individual in diet therapy must never be overlooked or minimized. Self-help is, of course, a very important component and the patient should clearly understand the vital need for intelligent co-operation on his part. The self-discipline necessary for the control of the appetite and the selection of the most suitable food must, in the last analysis depend on the individual's own initiative.

The increase in the number and variety of imported foods gives a wider choice of whole natural foods in and out of season. But the basic foods still remain and of these the whole grain foods are particularly important. Wheat, oats and rice form a substantial part of the daily diet. Bread, biscuits and other products should be made from wholewheat flour so as to contain the important fibre so lacking in white flour. Ideally, such bread should be home-made on the simple recipe advised by the vendors of the flour. Brown rice and oats are valuable foods but are, of course, rather starchy. However, they combine very well with the salad meals.

Breakfast Cereals

The breakfast cereals should be carefully chosen since they all do not come up to the standard of whole grains. Wholewheat and oat products are acceptable and a well-balanced muesli is to be recommended. As these are starchy foods they require thorough mastication. The addition of milk and sugar may not be a wise plan as the milk softens the cereals and permits swallowing without chewing and this may cause indigestion. It is better to eat them as dry as possible and sugar must be avoided (a little honey is preferable). These are the cold-weather foods which may be added to the fruits.

Meat

By far the majority of people partake of meat and fish and regard them as almost essential protein foods. As I have said, experience has shown that in the case of the sufferer from psoriasis, a low protein diet is preferable and that these foods should, therefore be excluded. For those who do not wish to go that far in changing their eating habits they should confine themselves to chicken and white fish. However, in using such foods two important points should be observed: First, they should be thoroughly cooked, and second, if reheated, you should make sure they are well heated right through.

Eggs

Eggs are of course protein foods and the sufferer should use them in moderation. They are a highly concentrated food with little or no fibre and should not be used more than three or four times in a week. They combine well with cooked vegetables, taking the usual place of meat or fish. They are rich in sulphur as shown by the discoloration they cause spoons and aluminium cooking vessels. They may be baked, boiled, poached or scrambled but should always be cooked slowly for ease of digestion.

Dairy Products

Dairy Products make a valuable contribution to nutrition. Milk should be regarded as a solid food and not merely as a drink. It combines well with fresh and dried fruit making a complete meal. It should be taken with a spoon or sipped slowly; hastily drank it may not curdle properly in the stomach making digestion more difficult. Fruit juices mixed with milk make the curdling process easier: pineapple juice used in this way quickly curdles the milk aiding in its digestion, beside being a very pleasant mixture.

Milk products form a substantial part of the vegetarian diet. Cheese, butter, cream, cottage cheese and yogurt in combination with fruit, salads and cooked vegetables can be relied on as an excellent source of nutrition. As a rich source of protein they should, of course, be used in moderation, but their inclusion in the diet helps avoid certain nutritional deficiencies (which is not to say that a vegan diet, which excludes these foods, cannot be nutritionally self-sufficient if properly arranged).

Hard cheese is a good food which can take the usual place of meat or fish in a meal. It is slow to digest but not indigestible, although when cooked digestion time is prolonged. Its protein value is high so that it should be used in moderation by those who may have to keep this part of food on the low side. It combines very well with fruit, salads and cooked vegetables (except potato) and is more easily digested in this way than when used with the carbohydrates. Butter and cream are possibly the most likeable of all fats, but they should be used sparingly, although when no other animal fat is included in the diet they may be used slightly more liberally. The unsalted form of butter is to be preferred when it is obtainable.

Cottage cheese and yogurt are two of the most useful and versatile of foods. Both may be used to supplement fruit and vegetable salads making a good combination for balanced nutrition. When using cottage cheese one should remember that it is a substitute for meat and adds essential calcium to the body. Yogurt is curdled milk containing lactic acid. It combines well with fruit and vegetable salads and used in that way is invaluable in restoring and maintaining the vital flora of the healthy bowel.

Beans, Peas and Lentils

While green beans and peas should be used as fresh vegetables the dried seeds of them, together with other pulses like lentils, make a valuable contribution to the menus. They are a mixture of protein and starchy elements and tend to make the system more alkaline. They need a good deal of preparation and cooking skill to make then usable; moderation in their use is called for with many people. They are best used in combination with the green salads, but used very sparingly at first. It must be said that with some people they appear to cause painful flatulence.

Nuts

The various nuts are protein foods, preferably used in the raw state. As they require thorough mastication, ineffective teeth or dentures may be a problem. The peanut is not, of course, a nut at all: it belongs to the legume family, but now is generally accepted and used as a nut. Roasted, it is palatable and makes a good food. It yields a very light oil that may be used as a dressing on salads. It is also made into peanut butter which, if carefully made and not over-salted, is a worthwhile addition to the menu. It is a protein food. In an analysis of it made some time ago Professor J. Russell Smith of Colombia University reported that 'it contains per pound more protein than a pound of sirloin steak, plus more carbohydrate than a pound of potatoes and one-third as much fat as a pound of butter.' It should be used in moderation.

Cooked Vegetables

The cooking of some vegetables is both necessary and desirable. It adds to their palatability and makes them more digestible. This is true of potatoes and other root vegetables. This applies also to beans and peas and to some leafy vegetables. But cooking also changes the nature of food and deprives it of some nutritional value. Cooked vegetables tend to undergo fermentation which gives rise to the feeling of fullness after such meals. Uncooked vegetables tend to check fermentation and do not promote fullness after meals. For this reason people may be under the wrong impression that cooked food is more nutritious than uncooked food, whereas in fact the opposite is true. Over-eating is also more likely to happen on cooked food.

To get the best value out of cooked vegetables, the cooking of them must be very carefully done. Boiling them in a generous amount of salted water and throwing away the liquid is just folly. If boiled, the least amount of water should be used and what remains of it used for soups or other such purposes. In other appropriate circumstances, they should be steamed, baked or pressure-cooked so as to preserve as much as possible their nutritional value and render them suitable for easy digestion. In passing, it might be pointed out that some vegetables, if obtained when young, like peas, may be eaten in their raw state; this applies also to the root vegetables which may be grated up and used in salads. Raw vegetables should be taken in smaller quantities than the cooked ones. For instance, a few fresh leaves of spinach may be used in salad, but one cannot imagine eating raw the amount of it that is pressed into the water of the saucepan for cooking!

Creating a Salad

The making of a salad that is pleasing to the eye, satisfying to taste and nutritious to the body is, perhaps, one of the highest achievements of the culinary art. There are many ingredients from which to choose. Lettuce, tomatoes and cucumber are possibly the limit for some people and indeed they do form the base of a good salad. But there are so many other vegetables that can be eaten raw and which should be added for their flavour and nutritional value. Leafy plants like watercress, mustard and cress, make excellent additions, together with radishes, spring onions and so on. The cabbage family may form the basis for a good salad, especially in winter time. The heart of it, shredded or finely chopped with tender sprouts of broccoli, cauliflower may all go into the salad bowl for the food values which they contain. The root vegetables, like carrots, parsnips, swede, artichokes and so on, when fresh and tender, may be grated up making many worthwhile additions, and sprigs of the various herbs may be added for their flavouring qualities

The bowl of salad may be made almost as interesting to the sight as the flower bowl and, if one has a garden, a few of the flower petals may be thrown in to heighten the colours. The dressing of the salad is important, adding to it flavour and nutritional value. Home-made mayonnaise is simple to make and serves a good purpose. A yolk of egg should be beaten slowly with drops of oil until it thickens, when lemon juice and sea salt may be added. A further spoonful of chopped parsley and onion will enhance the flavour and the value. A simpler dressing may be made of vegetable oil, lemon juice and sea salt to which a teaspoonful of chopped parsley and onion may be added. Whisk well or shake in a closed jar. Soya bean flour may be substituted for the egg and treated in the same manner, but it does not make quite so smooth a texture as the egg.

The fruit salad follows very much the same pattern as the vegetable one. The choice is just as large and should be exploited to the full. Apples, and the citrus fruits are with us all the year round so that they may well form the basis of such a salad. Of course, whenever a seasonal fruit comes on the market it should be included, especially the indigenous ones like strawberries, raspberries, cherries, gooseberries and so on. There is also a wide range of the dried fruits that may be used. Figs, dates, raisins and sultanas are welcome additions; soaking them in pineapple juice for a little time previously helps to sweeten the fresh fruits. As with the vegetable salad, the number of fruits are so numerous so that so many variations and combinations can be planned.

The dairy products should be used with the fruit salad. It makes an excellent combination for taste and nutrition. Cottage cheese, a good protein food which is more nutritious than meat, should be used in moderation. Cream, which brings out the delicate flavours of the fruit may be used occasionally. Ocassionally a change may be made using yogurt, a really good food for those who like its taste.

Soups

Soups should supplement salads. Many vegetables have outer parts that are not suitable for raw salads. Outside leaves of the cabbage family and the green tops of leeks are examples. They should not be discarded since they contain valuable food elements, particularly minerals. They should be put into a fairly large saucepan, together with several other root and leafy vegetables. Sprigs of various edible herbs should be added to enhance the flavour. The mixture should be cooked until the vegetables have been softened enough to be put through a blender, sieve or other suitable appliance. A little sea salt should be added.

This will provide one with a basic soup mixture that may be stored in the refrigerator and used from time to time. It can be flavoured and enriched in many ways. Tomato juice or *purée,* soya bean flour, oats, ground brown rice, yeast extract are all useful additions, and the enterprising person may think of other flavourings that may be employed to suit personal taste. Although we know that cooking deprives vegetables of some of their food value, a well-made soup retains as much of it as possible in the circumstances. Taken with wholewheat crackers or rye crispbread, soup forms a substantial part of a meal and is a very welcome hot dish in the winter time—which is not to say that it cannot be used in hot weather when it has been carefully chilled.

Drinks

Many different kinds of beverages are taken during the day, and although they are usually regarded as liquids they do, in fact, contain solid food elements. For instance, many people add sugar and milk to tea and coffee which belies the notion that they are liquid drinks. Indeed, in many cases, it is the sweetening that people crave for almost as much as for the tea or coffee. If they must be taken they should not be sweetened, they should be freshly made on the weak side, and not too close to a meal. People who have an abundance of fruit and vegetables in their diet have far less need and desire for beverages than those whose meals are largely made up of the rich protein and carbohydrate foods.

Fruit juices make excellent beverages and suit most people. Of course they have good food value, and contribute to the nutrition of the body. Drinks, hot or cold, made from lemon juice are particularly desirable, but water is the best and most natural drink. Of course, the chlorination of water may put people off drinking it unless something is added to mask the taste. Bottled spring water is available in most places, and if by its use one can develop the water-drinking habit, it will have been well worthwhile and in the interests of better health.

Summary
The psoriasis sufferer should carefully observe the foregoing notes about food and its use so that they become an integral part of his thinking about diet. It will help in the selection of the most suitable food, show how the best combinations can be made with it, and help to safeguard against future development of the complaint. It will be noted that emphasis has been laid on wholefoods rather than on the parts of them. This has been done in order to persuade the reader to use as great a variety of them as possible, particularly of the fruits and vegetables. I have found this in practice to be by far the better plan, far better than limiting the number and parts of foods and then trying to supplement them with the various parts that have been extracted from them. The thing to remember is that the food elements in a natural wholefood are well balanced, but all the necessary elements for a balanced nutrition is not contained in just one food. Therefore, the greater the diversity of them, the more certain it is that all the nutritional needs of the body will be satisfied.

5

MAKING DIET THERAPY EFFECTIVE

In an intractable complaint like psoriasis every effort must be made to make the treatment effective. This is particularly true of diet therapy. Just 'going on a diet' or 'dieting' may not be enough; other important factors, so closely related must be taken into consideration. The food may be good, adequate and properly balanced, but the patient may not be in a fit state to make full use of it. Obviously, it is not just a matter of taking food into the body: the body must be able to use it to its best advantage. In order to do so certain vital factors must be involved.

Nervous Energy and Stress
First of all, it needs nervous energy to efficiently carry out the processes of digestion, assimilation and elimination consequent upon the intake of food. The store of such energy depends upon the way a person lives. If a person is living beyond his physical, mental and emotional means that store of nervous energy will be dissipated to a point where all the functions in the body will be working below normal efficiency. Normal physical activity is necessary for the building up of nervous energy, but carried to excess will lead to its depletion. Working under strains of all kinds—worry, anxiety, boredom—stretches the

nervous system beyond its normal capacity, and may result in chronic fatigue.

The same is equally true of the stresses and strains of a mental or emotional nature. The strenuous pace of modern life imposes strains on the individual which he may find difficult to bear and he seeks relief in drug therapy. This is clearly shown by the millions of prescriptions that are written annually for such drugs as tranquillizers. The fact is that more visits are made to doctors' consulting rooms for stress disorders, and the ills and tensions that are the result of them, than for any other complaint. All this means is that the vital nervous energy has been drained to a point where the individual is suffering from a low grade of health, with few of the functions of the body performing efficiently, and with symptoms of lassitude, fatigue and depression.

We may be sure that the psoriasis sufferer, will also suffer from the stress which is a consequence of the burden of the complaint, not to mention the burden of the complaint itself. This will lead to a lowering of the nervous energy of the system with its adverse effects upon all the functions of the body and the usual malaise that goes with it. In such circumstances, the digestive and eliminative systems will not function efficiently. Of course food is necessary at such a time, but no one can expect that the individual will derive anything like the full benefit from it. We get energy from food, but we must remember that we use up nervous energy in doing so. So that in the last analysis it is the state of the nervous system that determines whether food is properly used within the body, and whether, of course, diet therapy will be effective.

Replacing Lost Energy

In so many cases there is a real need to rectify the strains which deplete the nervous energy. Experience has shown that the sufferer should give thought to the need for more sleep, rest and relaxation. Sufferers from skin complaints are liable to be plagued with disturbed sleep. Even the warmth of the bed may seem to act as an irritant making restful sleep difficult to obtain. Sleep is, of course, Nature's provision for the rebuilding of the nervous energy that is lost during the activities of daily life, and nothing undermines the digestive capacity more thoroughly than broken sleep.

A person so afflicted may resort to sleeping pills, but here again it is the digestive system that will suffer their side-effects. Nor will such sleep allow the mind and body to recuperate as in normal sleep. The sufferer should look to possible causes like the excessive use of stimulants such as tea and coffee, and the need for more relaxation. Fatigue and late hours may have been the starting point for the habit, and it is worth remembering that sleep before midnight pays off in more restful sleep.

The tense person cannot expect to make the best use of food. The constant leakage of the vital nervous energy will weaken the recuperative and curative power of the body, and lessen the effectiveness of food in reinforcing this power. The individual must see the need to relax and be willing to enforce it upon himself: to realize that the wastage of nervous energy serves no useful purpose and that it leads only to further problems.

It cannot be stressed too strongly that while the diet therapy outlined in the foregoing pages will greatly aid the operation of the natural healing power of the human body, and is, indeed, the only truly natural curative agency, it is only reasonable to expect the sufferer to aid Nature by getting proper sleep, rest and relaxation.